OSTEOPOROSIS DIET COOKBOOK FOR SENIORS

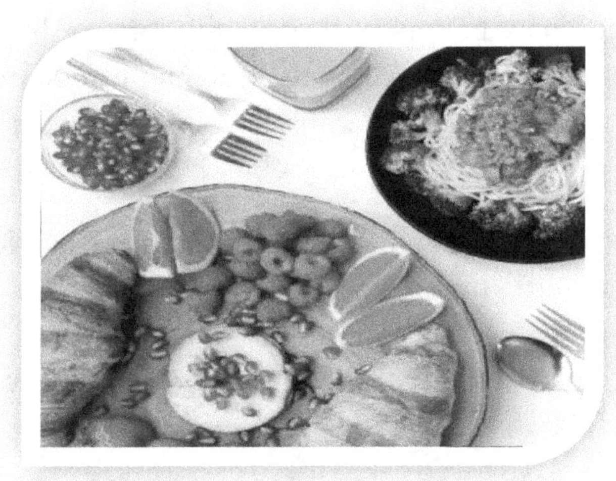

Nutrient-dense and Calcium-rich recipes guide for healthy bones

DR.CATHERINE THOMAS

TABLE OF CONTENT

CONCLUSION _____________________________________ **115**

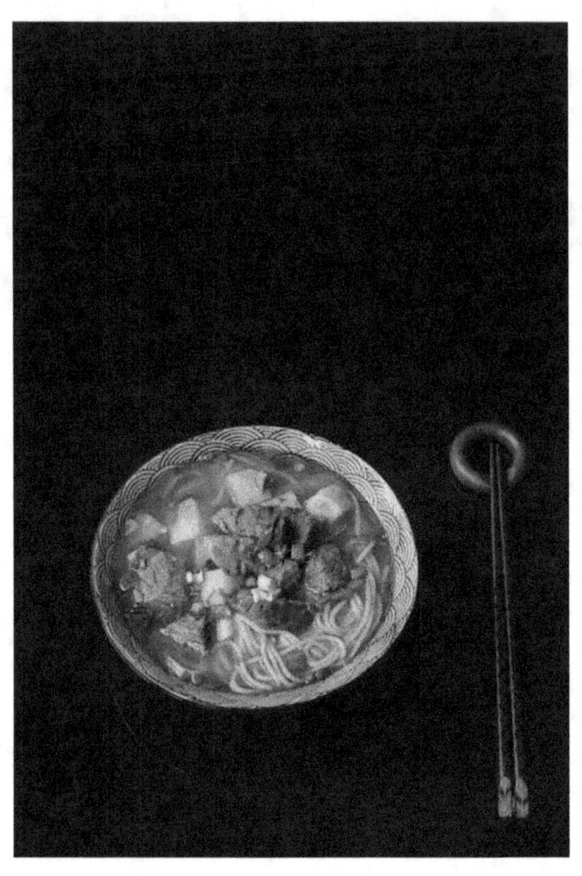

Welcome to the "Osteoporosis Diet Cookbook for Seniors," a comprehensive guide designed to empower you with the knowledge and recipes to naturally combat osteoporosis and enhance your overall health. As a nutritionist with years of experience, I understand the challenges that come with managing osteoporosis. This cookbook is crafted with your needs in mind, offering a collection of nutritious and flavorful anti-inflammatory recipes that not only support bone health but also delight your taste buds.

Osteoporosis is a condition that can significantly impact your quality of life, but with the right diet and lifestyle changes, you can take control of your health and well-being. Each recipe in this cookbook is thoughtfully created to provide essential nutrients, promote bone strength, and reduce inflammation. From hearty breakfasts to satisfying dinners and everything in between, you'll find a variety of delicious options to keep your meals exciting and beneficial.

Join me on this journey to better health, where every meal is an opportunity to nourish your body and support your bones. Together, we can make a positive impact on your life, one flavorful bite at a time.

In every sunrise, there's a chance to start anew,
A path to strength, where hope comes through.

With each meal prepared, with love and care,
You're building bones, so strong and rare.

Though osteoporosis may seem like a heavy plight,
You're not alone, we'll fight this fight.

With every bite of nutritious delight,
Your future's bright, your bones take flight.

Stay strong, dear friend, embrace each day,
With flavor and health, you'll find your way.

CHAPTER 1:

Understanding osteoporosis in seniors

Osteoporosis is a medical condition characterized by the weakening of bones, making them fragile and more prone to fractures. This condition is particularly prevalent among seniors, especially postmenopausal women, but it can affect older men as well. Understanding osteoporosis, its types, causes, symptoms, and preventive measures is crucial for seniors to manage and mitigate its effects on their health and quality of life.

Types of osteoporosis

1. **Primary Osteoporosis:**

    I. **Postmenopausal Osteoporosis:** This type occurs in women after menopause due to a significant drop in estrogen levels, a hormone that helps protect bone density. It typically affects bones like the spine, hip, and wrist.

II. Senile Osteoporosis: This type occurs in both men and women over the age of 70 and is linked to the natural aging process. It often affects the cortical and trabecular bone, leading to fractures in the hip, spine, and other areas.

2. Secondary Osteoporosis: This type results from medical conditions or medications that interfere with bone formation. Conditions such as hyperthyroidism, rheumatoid arthritis, and chronic kidney disease, as well as long-term use of corticosteroids, can lead to secondary osteoporosis.

Causes of osteoporosis

Osteoporosis develops when bone resorption (breakdown) exceeds bone formation, leading to a reduction in bone density. Several factors contribute to this imbalance:

1. Age: As people age, bone mass naturally decreases. The rate of bone loss accelerates in women after menopause and in men after the age of 70.

2. **Hormonal Changes:** In women, reduced estrogen levels post-menopause significantly impact bone density. In men, decreased testosterone levels can also contribute to bone loss.

3. **Genetics:** A family history of osteoporosis can increase the risk of developing the condition. Specific genetic factors affect bone mass and bone turnover.

4. **Nutritional Deficiencies:** Lack of essential nutrients like calcium and vitamin D, which are critical for bone health, can lead to weakened bones. Poor dietary habits throughout life can exacerbate this risk.

5. **Physical Inactivity:** Sedentary lifestyles contribute to bone loss. Weight-bearing and muscle-strengthening exercises are crucial for maintaining bone density.

6. **Medications and Medical Conditions:** Long-term use of corticosteroids, anticonvulsants, and certain other medications can lead to bone loss. Conditions like celiac disease, inflammatory bowel disease, and hyperthyroidism also affect bone health.

Symptoms of osteoporosis

Osteoporosis is often called the "silent disease" because it progresses without symptoms until a fracture occurs. However, there are some signs and symptoms that may indicate its presence:

1. **Fractures**: The most common and serious symptom. Fractures often occur in the hip, spine, or wrist, sometimes resulting from minor falls or even everyday activities.

2. **Back Pain**: Caused by fractures or collapsed vertebrae. This pain can be sudden and severe or chronic and dull.

3. **Loss of Height**: Over time, osteoporosis can cause a person to lose height due to compression fractures in the spine.

4. **Stooped Posture**: Also known as kyphosis or a dowager's hump, this occurs due to vertebral fractures leading to a curvature of the upper back.

Preventive measures for osteoporosis

Preventing osteoporosis involves a combination of lifestyle changes, dietary adjustments, and sometimes medical interventions. Here are key strategies to help prevent and manage osteoporosis:

1. **Adequate Calcium Intake:**

    I. Calcium is essential for bone health. Seniors should aim for at least 1,200 mg of calcium per day. Dairy products, leafy green vegetables, and fortified foods are good sources.

2. **Vitamin D:**

    I. Vitamin D helps the body absorb calcium. Seniors should ensure they get enough vitamin D through sunlight exposure, diet, or supplements, aiming for 800 to 1,000 IU per day.

3. **Balanced Diet:**

    I. A diet rich in fruits, vegetables, lean proteins,

II.   and whole grains supports overall health and provides essential nutrients for bone health.

4. **Regular Exercise:**

   I.   Weight-bearing exercises (like walking, jogging, and dancing) and muscle-strengthening exercises (like lifting weights) help maintain bone density and strength. Balance exercises (like Tai Chi) can help prevent falls.

5. **Healthy Lifestyle Choices:**

   I.   Avoid smoking and limit alcohol consumption, as both can contribute to bone loss and increase the risk of fractures.

6. **Bone Density Testing:**

   I.   Seniors, especially women over 65 and men over 70, should have regular bone density tests (DEXA scans) to monitor bone health and detect osteoporosis early.

7. **Medications**:

    I. For those at high risk or already diagnosed with osteoporosis, medications like bisphosphonates, hormone replacement therapy, and other bone-strengthening drugs may be prescribed by a healthcare provider.

8. **Fall Prevention**:

    I. Reducing the risk of falls is crucial for seniors with osteoporosis. This includes making homes safer (e.g., removing trip hazards, using grab bars), wearing supportive footwear, and reviewing medications that may affect balance.

Osteoporosis is a significant health concern for seniors, but with awareness and proactive measures, it is manageable. By understanding the types, causes, symptoms, and preventive strategies, seniors can take steps to protect their bone health and maintain a high quality of life. Through a combination of proper nutrition, regular exercise, and medical guidance, the impact of osteoporosis can be significantly reduced, allowing seniors to live active and fulfilling lives.

Impact of Osteoporosis on Senior Health

Osteoporosis significantly affects senior health, leading to various physical, emotional, and economic consequences. Understanding these impacts is crucial for both individuals and healthcare providers to effectively manage and mitigate the effects of this condition. Here are the primary ways osteoporosis impacts senior health:

1. Increased Fracture Risk

Fractures: Osteoporosis makes bones brittle and more susceptible to fractures, even from minor falls or stresses. The most common fracture sites are the hip, spine, and wrist.

- Hip Fractures: Often require surgical intervention and lengthy rehabilitation. Hip fractures can severely limit mobility and independence, and are associated with increased mortality rates among seniors.

- Vertebral Fractures: These can cause severe back pain, height loss, and deformities such as a stooped posture (kyphosis).

Vertebral fractures can also compress internal organs, leading to respiratory and digestive issues.

- **Wrist Fractures**: Can impair the ability to perform daily tasks and affect overall quality of life.

2. Decreased Mobility and Independence

Reduced Mobility: Fractures, particularly hip and spine fractures, often result in prolonged immobility and loss of function. This can lead to muscle atrophy, joint stiffness, and further decline in physical health.

Loss of Independence: Seniors with severe osteoporosis may require assistance with daily activities or need to move to assisted living facilities, significantly impacting their autonomy and quality of life.

3. Chronic Pain and Discomfort

Persistent Pain: Osteoporosis-related fractures can cause chronic pain, particularly in the back and hips. This persistent discomfort can affect sleep, mood, and overall well-being.

Pain Management: Chronic pain may necessitate long-term use of pain medications, which can have side effects and complicate other health conditions.

4. Psychological Impact

Emotional Distress: Living with osteoporosis and the fear of fractures can lead to anxiety and depression. The loss of independence and chronic pain further contribute to mental health challenges.

Social Isolation: Reduced mobility and the inability to participate in social activities can lead to feelings of isolation and loneliness, exacerbating mental health issues.

5. Economic Burden

Medical Costs: The treatment of fractures, including surgeries, hospital stays, rehabilitation, and ongoing medical care, imposes a significant financial burden on individuals and healthcare systems.

Indirect Costs: Loss of income for those who may still be working, as well as the cost of long-term care and assistance, add to the economic impact of osteoporosis.

6. Complications and Comorbidities

Complications: Seniors with osteoporosis are at higher risk for complications such as deep vein thrombosis (DVT) and pulmonary embolism (PE) due to prolonged immobility after fractures.

Comorbidities: Osteoporosis often coexists with other chronic conditions such as arthritis, diabetes, and cardiovascular disease, complicating management and treatment.

7. Quality of Life

Reduced Quality of Life: The combined effects of pain, reduced mobility, emotional distress, and financial burden significantly diminish the overall quality of life for seniors with osteoporosis.

Holistic Impact: The holistic impact on physical, emotional, and social well-being underscores the need for comprehensive management strategies that address all aspects of health.

The impact of osteoporosis on senior health is multifaceted and profound. It encompasses physical injuries, chronic pain, emotional distress, economic costs, and a substantial decrease in quality of life.

Addressing these impacts requires a proactive approach that includes prevention, early detection, effective treatment, and comprehensive support systems. By adopting a holistic approach to osteoporosis management, seniors can mitigate these effects and maintain a better quality of life.

Impact of Osteoporosis on Senior Health

Osteoporosis significantly affects senior health, leading to various physical, emotional, and economic consequences. Understanding these impacts is crucial for both individuals and healthcare providers to effectively manage and mitigate the effects of this condition. Here are the primary ways osteoporosis impacts senior health:

1. Increased Fracture Risk

Fractures: Osteoporosis makes bones brittle and more susceptible to fractures, even from minor falls or stresses. The most common fracture sites are the hip, spine, and wrist.

Hip Fractures: Often require surgical intervention and lengthy rehabilitation.

Hip fractures can severely limit mobility and independence, and are associated with increased mortality rates among seniors.

Vertebral Fractures: These can cause severe back pain, height loss, and deformities such as a stooped posture (kyphosis). Vertebral fractures can also compress internal organs, leading to respiratory and digestive issues.

Wrist Fractures: Can impair the ability to perform daily tasks and affect overall quality of life.

2. Decreased Mobility and Independence

Reduced Mobility: Fractures, particularly hip and spine fractures, often result in prolonged immobility and loss of function. This can lead to muscle atrophy, joint stiffness, and further decline in physical health.

Loss of Independence: Seniors with severe osteoporosis may require assistance with daily activities or need to move to assisted living facilities, significantly impacting their autonomy and quality of life.

3. Chronic Pain and Discomfort

Persistent Pain: Osteoporosis-related fractures can cause chronic pain, particularly in the back and hips. This persistent discomfort can affect sleep, mood, and overall well-being.

Pain Management: Chronic pain may necessitate long-term use of pain medications, which can have side effects and complicate other health conditions.

4. Psychological Impact

Emotional Distress: Living with osteoporosis and the fear of fractures can lead to anxiety and depression. The loss of independence and chronic pain further contribute to mental health challenges.

Social Isolation: Reduced mobility and the inability to participate in social activities can lead to feelings of isolation and loneliness, exacerbating mental health issues.

5. Economic Burden

Medical Costs: The treatment of fractures, including surgeries, hospital stays, rehabilitation, and ongoing medical care, imposes a significant financial burden on individuals and healthcare systems.

Indirect Costs: Loss of income for those who may still be working, as well as the cost of long-term care and assistance, add to the economic impact of osteoporosis.

6. Complications and Comorbidities

Complications: Seniors with osteoporosis are at higher risk for complications such as deep vein thrombosis (DVT) and pulmonary embolism (PE) due to prolonged immobility after fractures.

Comorbidities: Osteoporosis often coexists with other chronic conditions such as arthritis, diabetes, and cardiovascular disease, complicating management and treatment.

7. Quality of Life

Reduced Quality of Life: The combined effects of pain, reduced mobility, emotional distress, and financial burden significantly diminish the overall quality of life for seniors with osteoporosis.

Holistic Impact: The holistic impact on physical, emotional, and social well-being underscores the need for comprehensive management strategies that address all aspects of health.

The impact of osteoporosis on senior health is multifaceted and profound. It encompasses physical injuries, chronic pain, emotional distress, economic costs, and a substantial decrease in quality of life. Addressing these impacts requires a proactive approach that includes prevention, early detection, effective treatment, and comprehensive support systems. By adopting a holistic approach to osteoporosis management, seniors can mitigate these effects and maintain a better quality of life

Identifying Risk Factors of Osteoporosis for Seniors

Osteoporosis is a condition that primarily affects seniors, leading to weakened bones and an increased risk of fractures. Understanding the risk factors is crucial for prevention and early intervention. Here are the key risk factors for osteoporosis in seniors:

1. Age

> **Natural Bone Loss:** Bone density decreases with age. Seniors, particularly those over 65, are at higher risk because the body's ability to regenerate bone slows down.

2. Gender

Women: Women are more susceptible to osteoporosis, especially postmenopausal women, due to the rapid decline in estrogen levels, which are crucial for maintaining bone density.

Men: Although men have a higher peak bone mass, they still experience bone loss with age, and lower testosterone levels contribute to this risk.

3. Family History and Genetics

Genetic Predisposition: A family history of osteoporosis or fractures significantly increases the risk. Genetic factors influence bone density and the rate of bone loss.

4. Nutritional Factors

Calcium Deficiency: Inadequate intake of calcium throughout life can lead to reduced bone density. Calcium is vital for bone health.

Vitamin D Deficiency: Vitamin D is essential for calcium absorption. Low levels can result in decreased bone density and increased fracture risk.

Poor Nutrition: Diets low in essential nutrients, such as magnesium, phosphorus, and protein, contribute to weaker bones.

5. Physical Inactivity

Sedentary Lifestyle: Lack of weight-bearing and muscle-strengthening exercises accelerates bone loss. Regular physical activity is necessary to maintain bone strength.

6. Medical Conditions

Endocrine Disorders: Conditions like hyperthyroidism, hyperparathyroidism, and diabetes can affect bone metabolism.

Gastrointestinal Disorders: Diseases such as celiac disease, inflammatory bowel disease, and gastric bypass surgery can interfere with nutrient absorption, including calcium and vitamin D.

Chronic Kidney Disease: Impaired kidney function affects calcium and phosphate balance, leading to bone loss.

7. Medications

Corticosteroids: Long-term use of corticosteroids (e.g., prednisone) is a significant risk factor for osteoporosis as they interfere with bone rebuilding.

Anticonvulsants: Medications used to treat epilepsy can affect bone density.

Proton Pump Inhibitors: Long-term use can reduce calcium absorption.

8. Hormonal Changes

Menopause: The decrease in estrogen levels during menopause accelerates bone loss. Women who undergo early menopause or have their ovaries removed are at higher risk.

Low Testosterone in Men: Reduced testosterone levels in older men can contribute to bone loss.

9. Lifestyle Factors

Smoking: Tobacco use is linked to decreased bone density. It affects hormone levels and calcium absorption.

Alcohol Consumption: Excessive alcohol intake interferes with the balance of calcium and the production of bone-forming cells.

Caffeine and Soda: High consumption can lead to calcium loss through urine.

10. Body Weight and Build

Low Body Weight: Individuals with a low body mass index (BMI) have less bone mass to draw from as they age.

Small Frame Size: Those with a smaller body frame have less bone mass overall.

Identifying and understanding the risk factors for osteoporosis in seniors is critical for prevention and management. While some risk factors, such as age and genetics, cannot be changed, many lifestyle-related factors can be addressed through diet, exercise, and medical management. Seniors should be proactive in maintaining bone health by ensuring adequate nutrition, staying physically active, avoiding smoking and excessive alcohol consumption, and seeking medical advice for conditions or medications that may affect bone density. By managing these risk factors, the onset and progression of osteoporosis can be mitigated, enhancing the quality of life for seniors.

CHAPTER 2

Nutritional Guide to Build a Healthy Bone

The Role of Calcium in Bone Health for Seniors with Osteoporosis

Calcium is a critical mineral for maintaining bone health, particularly for seniors with osteoporosis. As a key component of bone tissue, calcium plays several essential roles in ensuring the integrity and strength of bones. Here's an in-depth look at the role of calcium in bone health for seniors with osteoporosis:

1. Bone Formation and Maintenance

Bone Mineralization: Calcium is the primary mineral found in bones, contributing to their hardness and strength. It combines with phosphate to form hydroxyapatite, the mineral complex that gives bones their rigidity.

Bone Remodeling: Throughout life, bones undergo continuous remodeling—a process where old bone tissue is replaced by new bone tissue. Adequate calcium intake is crucial to ensure that new bone formation keeps pace with bone resorption (breakdown).

2. Preventing Bone Loss

Calcium Deficiency and Bone Resorption: When dietary calcium is insufficient, the body compensates by resorbing calcium from the bones to maintain normal blood calcium levels, leading to bone loss.

Postmenopausal Bone Loss: In postmenopausal women, decreased estrogen levels accelerate bone resorption. Ensuring sufficient calcium intake can help mitigate this increased bone loss.

3. Supporting Bone Density

Bone Density Preservation: Adequate calcium intake helps maintain bone density, which is particularly important for seniors who are at higher risk of osteoporosis and fractures.

Bone Mass Accrual: While peak bone mass is typically achieved by early adulthood, maintaining adequate calcium levels throughout life helps preserve bone mass and prevent age-related declines.

4. Reducing Fracture Risk

Strengthening Bones: Stronger bones are less likely to fracture. Adequate calcium intake contributes to bone strength, reducing the likelihood of fractures from falls or minor injuries.

Enhancing Bone Quality: Calcium not only increases bone density but also improves the overall quality and resilience of bone tissue, making it more resistant to stress and impact.

5. Calcium in Diet and Supplementation

Dietary Sources: Seniors should consume calcium-rich foods such as dairy products (milk, yogurt, cheese), leafy green vegetables (kale, broccoli), fish with edible bones (sardines, salmon), and fortified foods (orange juice, cereals).

Supplements: When dietary intake is insufficient, calcium supplements can help meet the recommended daily intake. It's important to consult a healthcare provider to determine the appropriate dosage and type of supplement.

6. Synergistic Role with Vitamin D

Calcium Absorption: Vitamin D is essential for the efficient absorption of calcium from the digestive tract. Without adequate vitamin D, calcium cannot be effectively absorbed, regardless of dietary intake.

Bone Health Partnership: Together, calcium and vitamin D work synergistically to promote bone health. Vitamin D enhances calcium absorption and utilization, ensuring that sufficient calcium is available for bone formation and maintenance.

7. Recommended Calcium Intake for Seniors

Daily Requirements: The recommended daily intake of calcium for seniors is about 1,200 mg per day.

This can be achieved through a combination of diet and supplements if necessary.

Balancing Intake: It's important to balance calcium intake with other nutrients, such as magnesium and vitamin K, which also play roles in bone health. Over-supplementation should be avoided to prevent potential negative effects, such as kidney stones.

Calcium is indispensable for maintaining bone health in seniors with osteoporosis. Its roles in bone formation, maintenance, preventing bone loss, supporting bone density, and reducing fracture risk highlight its importance in managing osteoporosis. Seniors should focus on achieving adequate calcium intake through a balanced diet and, if necessary, supplements, while also ensuring sufficient vitamin D levels to enhance calcium absorption and utilization. By prioritizing calcium intake, seniors can better manage osteoporosis and maintain stronger, healthier bones.

Vitamins and Minerals for Bone Strength in Seniors with Osteoporosis

Maintaining bone strength is crucial for seniors, especially those with osteoporosis. While calcium is well-known for its role in bone health, several other vitamins and minerals are essential for optimal bone strength and overall skeletal health. Here are the key nutrients necessary for maintaining strong bones in seniors:

1. Calcium

Role: The primary mineral in bones, essential for bone formation and maintenance.

Sources: Dairy products (milk, cheese, yogurt), leafy green vegetables (kale, broccoli), fortified foods (orange juice, cereals), and fish with edible bones (sardines, salmon).

2. Vitamin D

Role: Enhances calcium absorption in the gut, regulates calcium levels in the blood, and promotes bone growth and remodeling.

Sources: Sun exposure, fatty fish (salmon, mackerel), fortified foods (milk, cereals), and supplements.

3. Magnesium

Role: Helps convert vitamin D into its active form, supports calcium metabolism, and is a component of the bone matrix.

Sources: Nuts (almonds, cashews), seeds (pumpkin, sunflower), whole grains, leafy green vegetables, and legumes.

4. Vitamin K

Role: Important for bone mineralization, helps bind calcium to the bone matrix, and activates proteins that regulate bone formation.

Sources: Leafy green vegetables (kale, spinach, broccoli), Brussels sprouts, and fermented foods (natto).

5. Phosphorus

Role: Works with calcium to build and maintain bones and teeth, and is a component of the bone mineral hydroxyapatite.

Sources: Dairy products, meat, fish, poultry, nuts, seeds, and whole grains.

6. Vitamin C

Role: Essential for collagen formation, which is a key component of the bone matrix. It also has antioxidant properties that protect bone cells.

Sources: Citrus fruits (oranges, grapefruits), strawberries, bell peppers, broccoli, and Brussels sprouts.

7. Vitamin A

Role: Necessary for bone growth and remodeling, helps regulate bone-building cells (osteoblasts) and bone-resorbing cells (osteoclasts).

Sources: Liver, fish oil, dairy products, and orange and yellow fruits and vegetables (carrots, sweet potatoes).

8. Zinc

Role: Supports bone formation and mineralization, and is involved in the synthesis of collagen.

: Meat, shellfish, legumes (chickpeas, lentils), seeds (pumpkin, sesame), and nuts (cashews, almonds).

9. B Vitamins

B6, B9 (Folate), and B12: These vitamins are essential for reducing homocysteine levels, which, when elevated, can be associated with bone loss and fractures.

Sources:

B6: Poultry, fish, potatoes, bananas, and chickpeas.

Folate: Leafy green vegetables, legumes, nuts, and fortified cereals.

B12: Meat, fish, dairy products, and fortified cereals.

10. Potassium

Role: Helps neutralize bone-depleting metabolic acids and reduces calcium loss in urine.

Sources: Bananas, potatoes, avocados, leafy greens, beans, and nuts.

11. Copper

Role: Important for the cross-linking of collagen fibers, which strengthens the bone matrix.

Sources: Shellfish, nuts, seeds, whole grains, and dark chocolate.

Practical Tips

1. **Balanced Diet**: Aim for a varied and balanced diet rich in the above vitamins and minerals. Include a variety of fruits, vegetables, lean proteins, and whole grains.

2. **Supplements**: If dietary intake is insufficient, consider supplements after consulting with a healthcare provider to determine appropriate types and dosages.

3. **Regular Check-Ups**: Regular bone density screenings and blood tests can help monitor bone health and nutrient levels.

4. **Sun Exposure**: Spend time outdoors to boost vitamin D levels naturally, but protect skin from excessive sun exposure.

5. Avoid Excesses: Limit intake of substances that can impair bone health, such as caffeine, alcohol, and high-sodium foods.

Ensuring adequate intake of essential vitamins and minerals is vital for seniors to maintain bone strength and combat osteoporosis.

By focusing on a nutrient-rich diet and considering supplementation when necessary, seniors can support their bone health and reduce the risk of fractures, thereby enhancing their overall quality of life.

Plant-Based Nutrients for Seniors with Osteoporosis

Incorporating plant-based nutrients into the diet is an excellent way for seniors with osteoporosis to maintain bone health. Plant-based diets are rich in vitamins, minerals, antioxidants, and other compounds that support bone strength and overall health. Here's how seniors can integrate these nutrients into their diets effectively:

1. Calcium-Rich Plant Foods

Sources:

Leafy Greens: Kale, bok choy, collard greens, and broccoli are excellent sources of calcium.

Fortified Foods: Plant-based milks (almond, soy, rice, oat) and orange juice often fortified with calcium.

Tofu and Tempeh: Made from soybeans, these are high in calcium, especially when prepared with calcium sulfate.

>**Almonds**: A good source of calcium, magnesium, and protein.

Tips:

Incorporate a variety of leafy greens in salads, soups, and smoothies.

Use fortified plant-based milk in cereals, smoothies, and cooking.

Add tofu and tempeh to stir-fries, salads, and sandwiches.

2. Vitamin D from Plant Sources

Sources:

Mushrooms: Certain types, like shiitake and maitake, can provide vitamin D when exposed to sunlight.

Fortified Foods: Plant-based milks and cereals are often fortified with vitamin D.

Tips:

Include mushrooms in meals, such as stir-fries, soups, and salads.

Ensure regular consumption of fortified plant-based milks and cereals.

3. Magnesium-Rich Foods

Sources:

Leafy Greens: Spinach, Swiss chard, and kale.

Nuts and Seeds: Pumpkin seeds, chia seeds, almonds, and cashews.

Legumes: Black beans, chickpeas, and lentils.

Whole Grains: Quinoa, brown rice, and whole wheat products.

Tips:

Add nuts and seeds to salads, yogurt, and oatmeal.

Incorporate legumes into soups, stews, and salads.

Use whole grains as a base for meals or side dishes.

4. Vitamin K from Plant Sources

Sources:

Leafy Greens: Kale, spinach, broccoli, and Brussels sprouts.

Fermented Foods: Natto (fermented soybeans) is particularly high in vitamin K2.

Tips:

Regularly include a variety of leafy greens in meals.

Explore fermented foods like natto, which can be added to salads or eaten with rice.

5. Phosphorus from Plant Sources

Sources:

Nuts and Seeds: Sunflower seeds, pumpkin seeds, and almonds.

Legumes: Lentils, chickpeas, and black beans.

Whole Grains: Brown rice, oats, and quinoa.

Tips:

Incorporate seeds into snacks and meals.

Use legumes as a protein source in various dishes.

Choose whole grains over refined grains for added nutrients.

6. Vitamin C for Collagen Production

Sources:

Citrus Fruits: Oranges, grapefruits, lemons, and limes.

Berries: Strawberries, blueberries, and raspberries.

Other Fruits and Vegetables: Kiwi, bell peppers, broccoli, and Brussels sprouts.

Tips:

Include a variety of fruits and vegetables in daily meals.

Use berries as a topping for cereals, yogurt, and desserts.

7. Vitamin A from Plant Sources

Sources:

Orange and Yellow Vegetables: Carrots, sweet potatoes, and pumpkins.

Leafy Greens: Spinach and kale.

Tips:

Include colorful vegetables in meals to ensure a variety of nutrients.

Use carrots and sweet potatoes in soups, stews, and roasted dishes.

8. Zinc from Plant Sources

Sources:

Legumes: Chickpeas, lentils, and beans.

Nuts and Seeds: Pumpkin seeds, sesame seeds, and cashews.

Whole Grains: Quinoa, oats, and whole wheat products.

Tips:

Include a variety of legumes, nuts, and seeds in your diet.

Opt for whole grain products to boost zinc intake.

9. B Vitamins for Bone Health

Sources:

Whole Grains: Brown rice, oats, and whole wheat products.

Legumes: Lentils, chickpeas, and black beans.

Nuts and Seeds: Almonds, sunflower seeds, and flaxseeds.

Leafy Greens: Spinach and kale.

Incorporate a range of whole grains in meals.

Add legumes to salads, soups, and casseroles.

Use nuts and seeds as snacks or meal toppings.

10. Potassium from Plant Sources

Sources:

Fruits: Bananas, avocados, and oranges.

Vegetables: Potatoes, sweet potatoes, and spinach.

Legumes: Beans and lentils.

Tips:

Include potassium-rich fruits and vegetables in your daily diet.

Use legumes as a regular part of your meals.

Practical Tips for Incorporating Plant-Based Nutrients

1. **Meal Planning:** Plan meals to include a variety of nutrient-rich plant foods. Focus on incorporating different colors and types of vegetables, fruits, legumes, nuts, seeds, and whole grains.

2. **Balanced Diet:** Ensure meals are well-balanced with a mix of macronutrients (proteins, fats, and carbohydrates) and micronutrients (vitamins and minerals).

3. **Snacking:** Choose healthy snacks like nuts, seeds, fruits, and vegetable sticks to boost nutrient intake throughout the day.

4. **Cooking Methods:** Use cooking methods that preserve nutrient content, such as steaming, roasting, and sautéing.

5. **Supplements:** Consider supplements if necessary, especially for nutrients like vitamin D, which may be difficult to obtain in sufficient quantities from plant sources alone.

Consult with a healthcare provider before starting any new supplement regimen.

Incorporating plant-based nutrients is an effective strategy for seniors with osteoporosis to maintain and enhance bone health. By focusing on a variety of nutrient-dense plant foods, seniors can ensure they receive essential vitamins and minerals that support strong bones and overall health. Making these dietary adjustments, along with regular physical activity and appropriate medical care, can help manage osteoporosis and improve quality of life.

<u>7-Days Meal Plan</u>

Day 1

Breakfast

- **Oatmeal** made with fortified almond milk, topped with **fresh berries**, **chia seeds**, and a drizzle of honey.

- **Orange juice** (fortified with calcium and vitamin D).

Snack

- **Almonds** and a small **apple**.

Lunch

- **Kale and tofu salad**: Massaged kale, grilled tofu, cherry tomatoes, cucumber, and carrots, dressed with olive oil and lemon.

- **Whole grain bread** slice.

Snack

- **Carrot sticks** with hummus.

Dinner

- **Baked salmon** (rich in vitamin D) with a side of **quinoa** and **steamed broccoli**.

- **Mixed greens salad** with olive oil and balsamic vinegar.

Day 2

Breakfast

- **Greek yogurt** parfait with **granola, flaxseeds,** and **blueberries.**

- **Green smoothie**: Spinach, banana, almond milk, and a scoop of protein powder.

Snack

- **Walnuts** and a small bunch of **grapes**.

Lunch

- **Lentil soup** with carrots, celery, and tomatoes.

- **Whole grain roll**.

Snack

- **Cucumber slices** with guacamole.

Dinner

- **Stuffed bell peppers**: Quinoa, black beans, corn, and spices, topped with avocado slices.

- **Steamed green beans.**

Breakfast

- **Scrambled eggs** with spinach and mushrooms, served with whole grain toast.

- **Fresh orange slices**.

Snack

- **Pumpkin seeds** and a small pear.

Lunch

- **Chickpea and avocado sandwich** on whole grain bread, with lettuce and tomato.

- **Side of baby carrots**.

Snack

- **Celery sticks** with almond butter.

Dinner

- **Grilled chicken breast** with a side of brown rice and roasted Brussels sprouts.

- **Mixed greens salad** with tomatoes, cucumbers, and olive oil dressing.

- **Smoothie bowl**: Blended banana, spinach, and fortified almond milk, topped with granola, chia seeds, and strawberries.

- **Herbal tea**.

- **Cashews** and an orange.

- **Quinoa salad**: Quinoa, black beans, corn, bell peppers, and avocado, with lime dressing.

- **Whole grain crackers**.

- **Red bell pepper slices** with hummus.

- **Baked cod** with a side of mashed sweet potatoes and steamed asparagus.

- **Leafy green salad** with olive oil and lemon dressing.

Breakfast

- **Whole grain pancakes** topped with **sliced bananas** and **a dollop of Greek yogurt.**

- **Fortified orange juice**.

Snack

- **Mixed nuts** and an apple.

Lunch

- **Tofu stir-fry**: Tofu, broccoli, bell peppers, snap peas, and carrots, served over brown rice.

- **Miso soup**.

Snack

- **Cherry tomatoes** with mozzarella balls.

Dinner

- **Grilled turkey burger** on a whole grain bun with lettuce, tomato, and avocado.

- **Sweet potato fries**.

Day 6

Breakfast

- **Greek yogurt** with honey, walnuts, and fresh raspberries.

- **Whole grain toast** with avocado.

Snack

- **Sunflower seeds** and a small apple.

Lunch

- **Spinach and chickpea curry** served over quinoa.

- **Cucumber salad** with dill and yogurt dressing.

Snack

- **Baby carrots** with hummus.

Dinner

- **Baked chicken breast** with a side of quinoa and roasted Brussels sprouts.

- **Mixed greens salad** with olive oil and balsamic vinegar.

Day 7

Breakfast

- **Smoothie**: Blended berries, spinach, fortified almond milk, and a scoop of protein powder.

- **Whole grain toast** with almond butter.

Snack

- **Almonds** and an orange.

Lunch

- **Lentil soup** with carrots, celery, and tomatoes.

- **Whole grain roll**.

Snack

- **Cucumber slices** with hummus.

Dinner

- **Grilled salmon** with a side of brown rice and steamed broccoli.

- **Mixed greens salad** with olive oil and lemon dressing.

CHAPTER 3

Breakfast:

| Calcium-Rich Oatmeal with Berries and Nuts |

Ingredients:

1 cup fortified almond milk

1/2 cup rolled oats

1/4 cup fresh blueberries

1/4 cup fresh strawberries, sliced

2 tbsp chopped almonds

1 tbsp chia seeds

1 tsp honey

Preparation:

1. In a small pot, bring almond milk to a boil.

2. Add oats and reduce heat to a simmer. Cook for 5-7 minutes, stirring occasionally.

3. Transfer oatmeal to a bowl and top with berries, almonds, chia seeds, and honey.

Nutritional Value (approx.):

Calories: 320

Protein: 9g

Calcium: 300mg

Vitamin D: 100 IUFiber: 8g

Cooking Time: 10 minutes

Spinach and Mushroom Scramble

Ingredients:

2 large eggs

1/2 cup fresh spinach, chopped

1/4 cup mushrooms, sliced

1 tbsp olive oil

Salt and pepper to taste

1 tbsp grated Parmesan cheese

Preparation:

1. Heat olive oil in a non-stick skillet over medium heat.

2. Add mushrooms and cook until tender, about 3-4 minutes.

3. Add spinach and cook until wilted, about 2 minutes.

4. Beat the eggs in a bowl, then pour into the skillet. Stir gently until eggs are fully cooked.

5. Season with salt and pepper, then sprinkle with Parmesan cheese.

Nutritional Value (approx.):

Calories: 230

Protein: 14g

Calcium: 150mg

Vitamin D: 40 IU

Fiber: 2g

Cooking Time: 10 minutes

Ingredients:

1 cup Greek yogurt (fortified with vitamin D)

1/2 cup granola

1/4 cup fresh raspberries

1/4 cup fresh blueberries

1 tbsp flaxseeds

1 tsp honey

Preparation:

1. In a glass or bowl, layer half of the Greek yogurt.

2. Add half of the granola, raspberries, and blueberries.

3. Repeat the layers with the remaining yogurt, granola, and fruit.

4. Sprinkle flaxseeds on top and drizzle with honey.

Nutritional Value (approx.):

Calories: 400

Protein: 18g

Calcium: 300mg

Vitamin D: 150 IU

Fiber: 7g

Cooking Time: 5 minutes

Avocado Toast with Tomato and Chia Seeds

Ingredients:

1 slice whole grain bread

1/2 ripe avocado

1/4 cup cherry tomatoes, halved

1 tbsp chia seeds

Salt and pepper to taste

1 tsp olive oil

Preparation:

1. Toast the whole grain bread.

2. Mash the avocado and spread it on the toast.

3. Top with cherry tomatoes, chia seeds, salt, and pepper.

4. Drizzle with olive oil.

Nutritional Value (approx.):

Calories: 300

Protein: 7g

Calcium: 100mg

Vitamin D: 0 IU

Fiber: 10g

Cooking Time: 5 minutes

Smoothie Bowl with Spinach and Banana

Ingredients:

1 cup fortified almond milk

1 banana

1 cup fresh spinach

1/2 cup frozen berries

1 tbsp almond butter

1 tbsp chia seeds

1 tbsp granola

Preparation:

1. Blend the almond milk, banana, spinach, frozen berries, and almond butter until smooth.

2. Pour the smoothie into a bowl.

3. Top with chia seeds and granola.

Nutritional Value (approx.):

Calories: 350

Protein: 10g

Calcium: 300mg

Vitamin D: 100 IU

Fiber: 8g

Cooking Time: 5 minutes

Ingredients:

1/2 block firm tofu, crumbled

1/4 cup red bell pepper, diced

1/4 cup onion, diced

1/2 cup fresh spinach, chopped

1 tbsp olive oil

1/2 tsp turmeric

Salt and pepper to taste

Preparation:

1. Heat olive oil in a skillet over medium heat.

2. Add onion and bell pepper, cook until tender, about 5 minutes.

3. Add crumbled tofu, turmeric, salt, and pepper. Cook for 5 minutes.

4. Stir in spinach and cook until wilted, about 2 minutes.

Cooking Time12 minutes

Nutritional Value (approx.):

Calories: 200

Protein: 14g

Calcium: 250mg

Vitamin D: 0 IU

Fiber: 4g

Cooking Time12 minutes

Chia Seed Pudding with Almond Milk and Berries

Ingredients:

1 cup fortified almond milk

1/4 cup chia seeds

1 tbsp honey

1/2 cup mixed berrie

Preparation:

1. Mix almond milk, chia seeds, and honey in a bowl.

2. Cover and refrigerate overnight.

3. Top with mixed berries before serving.

Cooking Time: 5 minutes (plus overnight refrigeration)

Nutritional Value (approx.):

Calories: 250

Protein: 7g

Calcium: 300mg

Vitamin D: 100 IU

Fiber: 10g

Cooking Time: 5 minutes (plus overnight refrigeration)

Ingredients:

1/2 cup cooked quinoa

1/4 cup almond milk (fortified)

1/4 cup fresh berries

1/4 apple, diced

2 tbsp chopped walnuts

1 tbsp honey

Preparation:

1. In a bowl, combine cooked quinoa and almond milk.

2. Top with berries, apple, walnuts, and honey.

Nutritional Value (approx.):

Calories: 350

Protein: 10g

Calcium: 150mg

Vitamin D: 50 IU

Fiber: 8g

Cooking Time:10 minutes (plus quinoa cooking time)

Sweet Potato and Black Bean Breakfast Burrito

Ingredients:

1 small sweet potato, diced

1/2 cup black beans, drained and rinsed

1/4 cup shredded cheese (fortified)

1 whole grain tortilla

1 tbsp olive oil

Salt and pepper to taste

Salsa for serving

Preparation:

1. Heat olive oil in a skillet over medium heat.

2. Add sweet potato and cook until tender, about 10 minutes.

3. Add black beans, salt, and pepper, and cook for 2-3 minutes.

4. Place the mixture in a tortilla, top with cheese, and roll up.

5. Serve with salsa.

Nutritional Value (approx.):

Calories: 400

Protein: 15g

Calcium: 200mg

Vitamin D: 100 IU

Fiber: 12g

Cooking Time: 15 minutes

Whole Grain Pancakes with Greek Yogurt and Fruit

Ingredients:

1 cup whole grain pancake mix

3/4 cup fortified almond milk

1 egg

1 tbsp olive oil

1/2 cup Greek yogurt (fortified)

1/2 cup fresh berries

1 tbsp honey

Preparation:

1. In a bowl, mix the pancake mix, almond milk, egg, and olive oil until smooth.

2. Heat a non-stick skillet over medium heat.

3. Pour 1/4 cup of batter for each pancake, cooking until bubbles form and edges are set, then flip and cook until golden brown.

4. Serve pancakes topped with Greek yogurt, berries, and honey.

Nutritional Value (approx.):

Calories: 450

Protein: 18g

Calcium: 300mg Vitamin D: 150 IU Fiber: 8g
Cooking Time:15 minutes

Kale and Quinoa Salad with Lemon-Tahini Dressing

Ingredients:

1 cup cooked quinoa

2 cups kale, chopped

1/2 cup cherry tomatoes, halved

1/4 cup red onion, thinly sliced

1/4 cup crumbled feta cheese

2 tbsp sunflower seeds

Dressing:

2 tbsp tahini

2 tbsp lemon juice

1 tbsp olive oil

1 tsp honey

Salt and pepper to taste

Preparation:

1. Massage kale with a small amount of olive oil until softened.

2. In a large bowl, combine quinoa, kale, cherry tomatoes, red onion, feta cheese, and sunflower seeds.

3. In a small bowl, whisk together tahini, lemon juice, olive oil, honey, salt, and pepper.

4. Drizzle the dressing over the salad and toss to coat.

Nutritional Value (approx.):

Calories: 350

Protein: 12g

Calcium: 150mg

Vitamin D: 0 IU

Fiber: 8g

Cooking Time: 15 minutes

Ingredients:

1 cup lentils, rinsed

1 cup fresh spinach, chopped

1 carrot, diced

1 celery stalk, diced

1 small onion, diced

2 garlic cloves, minced

1 tbsp olive oil

4 cups low-sodium vegetable broth

1 tsp cumin

1 tsp paprika

Salt and pepper to taste

Preparation:

1. Heat olive oil in a large pot over medium heat.

2. Add onion, carrot, celery, and garlic. Sauté until vegetables are softened, about 5 minutes.

3. Stir in cumin and paprika, then add lentils and vegetable broth. Bring to a boil.

4. Reduce heat and simmer for 25-30 minutes, or until lentils are tender.

5. Stir in spinach and cook until wilted, about 2 minutes. Season with salt and pepper.

Nutritional Value (approx.):

Calories: 250

Protein: 14g

Calcium: 100mg

Vitamin D: 0 IU

Fiber: 12g **Cooking Time: 35 minutes**

Grilled Chicken and Avocado Wrap

Ingredients:

1 whole grain tortilla

1/2 cup cooked, sliced chicken breast

1/4 avocado, sliced

1/4 cup shredded lettuce

1/4 cup diced tomatoes

1 tbsp Greek yogurt (fortified)

1 tbsp salsa

Preparation:

1. Warm the tortilla in a skillet or microwave.

2. Spread Greek yogurt and salsa over the tortilla.

3. Layer with chicken, avocado, lettuce, and tomatoes.

4. Roll up the tortilla tightly and slice in half.

Nutritional Value (approx.):

Calories: 350

Protein: 28g

Calcium: 150mg

Vitamin D: 40 IU

Fiber: 8g **Cooking Time: 10 minutes**

Chickpea and Avocado Salad

Ingredients:

1 can chickpeas, drained and rinsed

1 ripe avocado, diced

1/4 cup red bell pepper, diced

1/4 cup cucumber, diced

1/4 cup red onion, diced

2 tbsp chopped fresh parsley

1 tbsp lemon juice

1 tbsp olive oil

Salt and pepper to taste

Preparation:

1. In a large bowl, combine chickpeas, avocado, bell pepper, cucumber, red onion, and parsley.

2. Drizzle with lemon juice and olive oil. Season with salt and pepper.

3. Toss gently to combine.

Nutritional Value (approx.):

Calories: 300

Protein: 10g

Calcium: 80mg

Vitamin D: 0 IU

Fiber: 12g   **Cooking Time: 10 minutes**

Salmon and Spinach Salad

Ingredients:

1 cup fresh spinach

1/2 cup cooked salmon, flaked

1/4 cup cherry tomatoes, halved

1/4 cup cucumber, sliced

1/4 avocado, sliced

1 tbsp sunflower seeds

Dressing:

1 tbsp olive oil

1 tbsp lemon juice

1 tsp Dijon mustard

Salt and pepper to taste

Preparation:

1. In a large bowl, combine spinach, salmon, cherry tomatoes, cucumber, avocado, and sunflower seeds.

2. In a small bowl, whisk together olive oil, lemon juice, Dijon mustard, salt, and pepper.

3. Drizzle the dressing over the salad and toss to coat.

Nutritional Value (approx.):

Calories: 350

Protein: 20g

Calcium: 100mg

Vitamin D: 200 IU

Fiber: 6g

Cooking Time: 10 minutes

Ingredients:

2 bell peppers, halved and seeds removed

1 cup cooked quinoa

1/2 cup black beans, drained and rinsed

1/4 cup corn kernels

1/4 cup diced tomatoes

1/4 cup shredded cheese (fortified)

1 tsp cumin

1 tsp paprika

Salt and pepper to taste

Preparation:

1. Preheat the oven to 375°F (190°C).

2. In a large bowl, combine cooked quinoa, black beans, corn, diced tomatoes, cumin, paprika, salt, and pepper.

3. Stuff each bell pepper half with the quinoa mixture.

4. Place stuffed peppers in a baking dish and top with shredded cheese.

5. Bake for 25-30 minutes, until peppers are tender and cheese is melted.

Nutritional Value (approx.):

Calories: 300

Protein: 12g

Calcium: 150mg

Vitamin D: 100 IU

Fiber: 10g   **Cooking Time: 35 minutes**

Tofu and Vegetable Stir-Fry

Ingredients:

1/2 block firm tofu, cubed

1 cup broccoli florets

1/2 cup red bell pepper, sliced

1/2 cup snap peas

1 carrot, sliced

2 tbsp soy sauce

1 tbsp olive oil

1 tsp ginger, grated

1 garlic clove, minced

1 cup cooked brown rice

Preparation:

1. Heat olive oil in a large skillet or wok over medium-high heat.

2. Add garlic and ginger, sauté for 1 minute.

3. Add tofu and cook until golden brown, about 5 minutes.

4. Add broccoli, bell pepper, snap peas, and carrot. Cook until vegetables are tender-crisp, about 5-7 minutes.

5. Stir in soy sauce and cook for an additional 2 minutes.

6. Serve over cooked brown rice.

Nutritional Value (approx.):

Calories: 400

Protein: 18g

Calcium: 200mg

Vitamin D: 0 IU

Fiber: 10g   **Cooking Time: 20 minutes**

Sweet Potato and Black Bean Tacos

Ingredients:

1 medium sweet potato, peeled and diced

1/2 cup black beans, drained and rinsed

1/4 cup corn kernels

1/4 cup diced tomatoes

1 tbsp olive oil

1 tsp cumin

1 tsp paprika

Salt and pepper to taste

4 small corn tortillas

1/4 cup shredded cheese (fortified)

Preparation:

1. Preheat the oven to 400°F (200°C).

2. Toss diced sweet potato with olive oil, cumin, paprika, salt, and pepper. Spread on a baking sheet.

3. Roast for 20-25 minutes, until tender.

4. In a bowl, combine roasted sweet potato, black beans, corn, and diced tomatoes.

5. Warm tortillas and fill with the sweet potato mixture. Top with shredded cheese.

Nutritional Value (approx.):

Calories: 350

Protein: 12g

Calcium: 150mg

Vitamin D: 0 IU

Fiber: 10g

Cooking Time:30 minutes

Mediterranean Chickpea Salad

Ingredients:

1 can chickpeas, drained and rinsed

1/2 cup cherry tomatoes, halved

1/2 cucumber, diced

1/4 cup red onion, diced

1/4 cup Kalamata olives, sliced

1/4 cup feta cheese, crumbled

2 tbsp chopped fresh parsley

Dressing:

2 tbsp olive oil

1 tbsp red wine vinegar

1 tsp lemon juice

Salt and pepper to taste

Preparation:

1. In a large bowl, combine chickpeas, cherry tomatoes, cucumber, red onion, olives, feta cheese, and parsley.

2. In a small bowl, whisk together olive oil, red wine vinegar, lemon juice, salt, and pepper.

3. Drizzle the dressing over the salad and toss to coat.

Nutritional Value (approx.):

Calories: 300

Protein: 10g

Calcium: 150mg

Vitamin D: 0 IU

Fiber: 8g **Cooking Time: 10 minutes**

Turkey and Avocado Salad

Ingredients:

2 cups mixed greens

1/2 cup cooked turkey breast, sliced

1/2 avocado, sliced

1/4 cup cherry tomatoes, halved

1/4 cup cucumber, sliced

1 tbsp sunflower seeds

Dressing:

1 tbsp olive oil

1 tbsp balsamic vinegar

Salt and pepper to taste

Preparation:

1. In a large bowl, combine mixed greens, turkey, avocado, cherry tomatoes, cucumber, and sunflower seeds.

2. In a small bowl, whisk together olive oil, balsamic vinegar, salt, and pepper.

3. Drizzle the dressing over the salad and toss to coat.

Nutritional Value (approx.):

Calories: 350

Protein: 20g

Calcium: 100mg

Vitamin D: 0 IU

Fiber: 6g

Cooking Time: 10 minutes

Dinner:

Baked Salmon with Asparagus

Ingredients:

2 salmon fillets (about 6 oz each)

1 bunch asparagus, trimmed

1 tbsp olive oil

1 lemon, sliced

1 tsp dried dill

Salt and pepper to taste

Preparation:

1. Preheat the oven to 400°F (200°C).

2. Place salmon fillets and asparagus on a baking sheet.

3. Drizzle with olive oil, and season with dill, salt, and pepper.

4. Arrange lemon slices over the salmon.

5. Bake for 20 minutes, until salmon is cooked through and asparagus is tender.

Nutritional Value (approx.):

Calories: 400

Protein: 35g

Calcium: 60mg

Vitamin D: 600 IU

Fiber: 4g **Cooking Time: 25 minutes**

Quinoa and Black Bean Stuffed Bell Peppers

Ingredients:

4 bell peppers, halved and seeds removed

1 cup cooked quinoa

1 can black beans, drained and rinsed

1 cup corn kernels

1 cup diced tomatoes

1 tsp cumin

1 tsp chili powder

1 cup shredded cheese (fortified)

Salt and pepper to taste

Preparation:

1. Preheat the oven to 375°F (190°C).

2. In a large bowl, mix cooked quinoa, black beans, corn, diced tomatoes, cumin, chili powder, salt, and pepper.

3. Stuff bell pepper halves with the quinoa mixture.

4. Place stuffed peppers in a baking dish and top with shredded cheese.

5. Bake for 25-30 minutes, until peppers are tender and cheese is melted.

Nutritional Value (approx.):

Calories: 350

Protein: 15g

Calcium: 200mg

Vitamin D: 80 IU

Fiber: 10g **Cooking Time: 35 minutes**

Chicken and Broccoli Stir-Fry

Ingredients:

2 boneless, skinless chicken breasts, sliced

2 cups broccoli florets

1 red bell pepper, sliced

1 carrot, sliced

2 garlic cloves, minced

1 tbsp olive oil

2 tbsp soy sauce (low sodium)

1 tbsp honey

1 tsp grated ginger

Preparation:

1. Heat olive oil in a large skillet over medium-high heat.

2. Add garlic and ginger, sauté for 1 minute.

3. Add chicken and cook until browned, about 5-7 minutes.

4. Add broccoli, bell pepper, and carrot. Stir-fry for 5-7 minutes, until vegetables are tender-crisp.

5. Stir in soy sauce and honey, cook for an additional 2 minutes.

Nutritional Value (approx.):

Calories: 350

Protein: 30g

Calcium: 80mg

Vitamin D: 0 IU

Fiber: 6g   **Cooking Time: 20 minutes**

Spinach and Feta Stuffed Chicken Breast

Ingredients:

2 boneless, skinless chicken breasts

1 cup fresh spinach, chopped

1/4 cup crumbled feta cheese

1 tbsp olive oil

1 tsp garlic powder

Salt and pepper to taste

Cooking Time: 20 minutes

Preparation:

1. Preheat the oven to 375°F (190°C).

2. Slice a pocket into each chicken breast.

3. In a bowl, mix spinach and feta cheese.

4. Stuff the chicken breasts with the spinach mixture and secure with toothpicks.

5. Brush with olive oil and season with garlic powder, salt, and pepper.

6. Place in a baking dish and bake for 25-30 minutes, until chicken is cooked through.

Nutritional Value (approx.):

Calories: 300

Protein: 35g

Calcium: 150mg

Vitamin D: 0 IU

Fiber: 2g

Cooking Time: 35 minutes

Sweet Potato and Chickpea Curry

Ingredients:

1 large sweet potato, peeled and diced

1 can chickpeas, drained and rinsed

1 can coconut milk (light)

1 onion, diced

2 garlic cloves, minced

1 tbsp olive oil

1 tbsp curry powder

1 tsp cumin

1 cup spinach, chopped

Salt and pepper to taste **Cooking Time: 35 minutes**

Preparation:

1. Heat olive oil in a large pot over medium heat.

2. Add onion and garlic, sauté until softened, about 5 minutes.

3. Stir in curry powder and cumin, cook for 1 minute.

4. Add sweet potato, chickpeas, and coconut milk. Bring to a boil.

5. Reduce heat and simmer for 20-25 minutes, until sweet potatoes are tender.

6. Stir in spinach and cook until wilted, about 2 minutes. Season with salt and pepper.

Nutritional Value (approx.):

Calories: 350

Protein: 10g

Calcium: 100mg

Vitamin D: 0 IU

Fiber: 12g   **Cooking Time: 35 minutes**

Baked Cod with Garlic and Herbs

Ingredients:

2 cod fillets (about 6 oz each)

2 tbsp olive oil

2 garlic cloves, minced

1 lemon, sliced

1 tsp dried thyme

1 tsp dried parsley

Salt and pepper to taste

Preparation:

1. Preheat the oven to 375°F (190°C).

2. Place cod fillets in a baking dish.

3. Drizzle with olive oil and top with minced garlic, lemon slices, thyme, parsley, salt, and pepper.

4. Bake for 20-25 minutes, until fish is opaque and flakes easily with a fork.

Nutritional Value (approx.):

Calories: 250

Protein: 35g

Calcium: 40mg

Vitamin D: 300 IU

Fiber: 1g **Cooking Time: 30 minutes**

Mushroom and Spinach Risotto

Ingredients:

1 cup Arborio rice

1 cup fresh spinach, chopped

1 cup mushrooms, sliced

1 small onion, diced

2 garlic cloves, minced

1 tbsp olive oil

1/2 cup grated Parmesan cheese (fortified)

4 cups low-sodium chicken broth

1/2 cup white wine (optional)

Salt and pepper to taste

Preparation:

1. Heat olive oil in a large saucepan over medium heat.

2. Add onion and garlic, sauté until softened, about 5 minutes.

3. Add mushrooms and cook until tender, about 5 minutes.

4. Stir in Arborio rice and cook for 1 minute.

5. Add white wine and cook until absorbed (optional).

6. Gradually add chicken broth, 1 cup at a time, stirring frequently until absorbed.

7. Stir in spinach and Parmesan cheese, cook until spinach is wilted and cheese is melted. Season with salt and pepper.

Nutritional Value (approx.):

Calories: 400

Protein: 15g

Calcium: 200mg

Vitamin D: 0 IU

Fiber: 4g   **Cooking Time: 35 minutes**

Turkey Meatballs with Zucchini Noodles

Ingredients:

1 lb ground turkey

1/4 cup grated Parmesan cheese

1/4 cup breadcrumbs

1 egg, beaten

2 garlic cloves, minced

1 tsp dried oregano

1 tsp dried basil

2 tbsp olive oil

2 large zucchinis, spiralized

1 cup marinara sauce (low sodium)

Salt and pepper to taste

Preparation:

1. In a large bowl, mix ground turkey, Parmesan cheese, breadcrumbs, egg, garlic, oregano, basil, salt, and pepper.

2. Form into small meatballs.

3. Heat olive oil in a large skillet over medium heat. Cook meatballs until browned and cooked through, about 10 minutes.

4. Add marinara sauce to the skillet and simmer for 5 minutes.

5. Meanwhile, heat a separate skillet over medium heat and sauté zucchini noodles for 2-3 minutes.

6. Serve meatballs over zucchini noodles.

Nutritional Value (approx.):

Calories: 350

Protein: 25g

Calcium: 150mg

Vitamin D: 0 IU

Fiber: 5g   **Cooking Time: 20 minutes**

Vegetable and Tofu Stir-Fry

Ingredients:

1 block firm tofu, cubed

1 cup broccoli florets

1 red bell pepper, sliced

1 cup snap peas

1 carrot, sliced

2 garlic cloves, minced

1 tbsp olive oil

2 tbsp soy sauce (low sodium)

1 tsp sesame

1 tsp honey

Salt and pepper to taste

Cooked brown rice or quinoa for serving

Preparation:

1. Heat olive oil in a large skillet or wok over medium-high heat.

2. Add garlic and sauté for 1 minute.

3. Add tofu and cook until golden brown, about 5 minutes.

4. Add broccoli, bell pepper, snap peas, and carrot. Stir-fry for 5-7 minutes until vegetables are tender-crisp.

5. In a small bowl, whisk together soy sauce, sesame oil, honey, salt, and pepper.

6. Pour the sauce over the tofu and vegetables. Stir well to coat evenly.

7. Serve over cooked brown rice or quinoa.

Nutritional Value (approx.):

Calories: 400

Protein: 20g

Calcium: 100mg

Vitamin D: 0 IU

Fiber: 8g   **Cooking Time: 20 minutes**

Mediterranean Baked Chicken

Ingredients:

4 boneless, skinless chicken breasts

1/4 cup olive oil

2 tbsp lemon juice

2 tsp dried oregano

2 tsp dried basil

1 tsp garlic powder

Salt and pepper to taste

1/2 cup cherry tomatoes, halved

1/4 cup Kalamata olives, sliced

1/4 cup crumbled feta cheese

Fresh parsley for garnish

Preparation:

1. Preheat the oven to 375°F (190°C).

2. In a bowl, whisk together olive oil, lemon juice, oregano, basil, garlic powder, salt, and pepper.

3. Place chicken breasts in a baking dish and pour the marinade over them. Ensure chicken is coated evenly.

4. Scatter cherry tomatoes and olives around the chicken.

5. Bake for 25-30 minutes, or until chicken is cooked through.

6. Sprinkle feta cheese over the chicken during the last 5 minutes of baking.

7. Garnish with fresh parsley before serving.

Nutritional Value (approx.):

Calories: 300

Protein: 30g

Calcium: 80mg

Vitamin D: 0 IU

Fiber: 2g   **Cooking Time: 35 minutes**

Snacks and Dessert:

Greek Yogurt Parfait

Ingredients:

1 cup Greek yogurt (fortified)

1/2 cup mixed berries (blueberries, strawberries)

2 tbsp granola

1 tbsp honey

Preparation:

1. In a glass or bowl, layer Greek yogurt, mixed berries, and granola.

2. Drizzle honey on top.

3. Serve chilled.

Nutritional Value (approx.):

Calories: 200

Protein: 15g

Calcium: 250mg

Vitamin D: 0 IU

Fiber: 4g   **Preparation Time: 5 minutes**

Baked Apple with Cinnamon

Ingredients:

1 large apple, cored

1 tsp cinnamon

1 tbsp honey

1 tbsp chopped walnuts

Preparation:

1. Preheat the oven to 375°F (190°C).

2. Place the cored apple on a baking sheet.

3. Sprinkle cinnamon over the apple and drizzle with honey.

4. Bake for 20-25 minutes, until apple is tender.

5. Sprinkle chopped walnuts on top before serving.

Nutritional Value (approx.):

Calories: 150

Protein: 2g

Calcium: 20mg

Vitamin D: 0 IU

Fiber: 4g   **Cooking Time: 25 minutes**

Dark Chocolate-Dipped Strawberries

Ingredients:

1/2 cup dark chocolate chips (70% cocoa or higher)

10 fresh strawberries, washed and dried

Preparation:

1. Melt dark chocolate chips in a microwave-safe bowl in 30-second intervals, stirring until smooth.

2. Dip each strawberry into the melted chocolate, coating halfway.

3. Place dipped strawberries on a parchment-lined tray.

4. Refrigerate for 15-20 minutes to set the chocolate.

Nutritional Value (approx. per serving of 2 strawberries):

Calories: 80

Protein: 1g

Calcium: 20mg

Vitamin D: 0 IU

Fiber: 2g   **Preparation Time: 15 minutes**

Frozen Banana Bites

Ingredients:

2 ripe bananas, peeled and sliced into rounds

1/4 cup almond butter

1/4 cup dark chocolate chips

1 tbsp coconut oil

Preparation:

1. Spread almond butter on half of the banana slices and top with the remaining slices to make sandwiches.

2. Place banana sandwiches on a parchment-lined tray and freeze for 1 hour.

3. In a microwave-safe bowl, melt dark chocolate chips with coconut oil in 30-second intervals, stirring until smooth.

4. Dip each frozen banana sandwich into the melted chocolate, coating halfway.

5. Return coated banana bites to the freezer for another 30 minutes to set.

Nutritional Value (approx. per serving of 2 banana bites):

Calories: 150

Protein: 2g

Calcium: 10mg

Vitamin D: 0 IU

Fiber: 3g   **Preparation Time: 90 minutes (including freezing time)**

Chia Seed Pudding

Ingredients:

2 tbsp chia seeds

1/2 cup almond milk (fortified)

1/2 tsp vanilla extract

1 tbsp maple syrup

Fresh fruit for topping (e.g., berries, sliced banana)

Preparation:

1. In a bowl, mix chia seeds, almond milk, vanilla extract, and maple syrup.

2. Stir well to combine and let sit for 10 minutes.

3. Stir again to prevent clumping and refrigerate for at least 2 hours or overnight.

4. Top with fresh fruit before serving.

Nutritional Value (approx. per serving):

Calories: 150

Protein: 3g

Calcium: 150mg

Vitamin D: 0 IU

Fiber: 8g **Preparation Time: 10 minutes (plus chilling time)**

Almonds and Dried Fruit Mix

Ingredients:

1/4 cup almonds

1/4 cup dried apricots, chopped

1/4 cup dried cranberries

Preparation:

1. Mix almonds, dried apricots, and dried cranberries in a bowl.

2. Serve as a snack mix.

Nutritional Value (approx. per serving):

Calories: 150

Protein: 4g

Calcium: 50mg

Vitamin D: 0 IU

Fiber: 3g **Preparation Time: 2 minutes**

Ingredients:

1/2 cup low-fat cottage cheese

1/2 cup fresh pineapple chunks

Preparation:

1. Spoon cottage cheese into a bowl.

2. Top with fresh pineapple chunks.

Nutritional Value (approx. per serving):

Calories: 100

Protein: 12g

Calcium: 100mg

Vitamin D: 0 IU

Fiber: 1g

Preparation Time: 2 minutes

Whole Grain Crackers with Hummus

Ingredients:

4 whole grain crackers

2 tbsp hummus (flavored or plain)

Preparation:

1. Spread hummus on each whole grain cracker.

2. Serve as a snack.

Nutritional Value (approx. per serving):

Calories: 100

Protein: 3g

Calcium: 20mg

Vitamin D: 0 IU

Fiber: 2g

Preparation Time: 2 minutes

Ingredients:

1 cup edamame (shelled)

Sea salt (optional)

Preparation:

1. Steam or boil edamame until tender, about 5-7 minutes.

2. Drain and sprinkle with sea salt if desired.

3. Serve as a snack.

Nutritional Value (approx. per serving):

Calories: 120

Protein: 11g

Calcium: 100mg

Vitamin D: 0 IU

Fiber: 6g

Preparation Time: 10 minutes

Yogurt-Covered Almonds

Ingredients:

1/2 cup whole almonds

1/4 cup Greek yogurt (fortified)

1 tsp honey

Preparation:

1. Mix Greek yogurt and honey in a bowl.

2. Dip each almond into the yogurt mixture to coat.

3. Place coated almonds on a parchment-lined tray and freeze for 1 hour.

Preparation Time: 10 minutes

CONCLUSION

In concluding this osteoporosis diet cookbook for seniors, it's crucial to emphasize the transformative power of nutrition in enhancing bone health and overall well-being. By incorporating these nutrient-dense recipes rich in calcium, vitamin D, and other essential nutrients, seniors can proactively combat osteoporosis and improve their quality of life.

The journey to optimal health is not just about what we eat but how we nourish our bodies. This cookbook goes beyond providing recipes; it's a guide to creating a lifestyle rooted in wholesome, flavorful, and anti-inflammatory foods. Each dish is crafted with care to offer not only nutritional benefits but also culinary delight, ensuring that eating well becomes a joyful experience.

Remember, health is a journey, and every step counts. As you embark on this osteoporosis-friendly diet, let it be a reminder that small changes can yield significant results. Empower yourself with the knowledge and tools provided in this cookbook to make informed choices and prioritize your well-being.

So, embrace this journey with enthusiasm and dedication. Let each meal be a celebration of vitality and strength. Your health is your greatest asset, and by nourishing your body with love and intention, you're laying the foundation for a vibrant and fulfilling life. Cheers to good health and delicious meals.

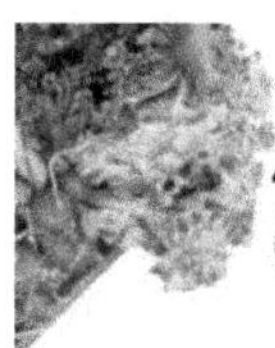

WEEKLY MEAL PLANNER

MONDAY	BREAKFAST	
	LUNCH	
	DINNER	
TUESDAY	BREAKFAST	
	LUNCH	
	DINNER	
WEDNESDAY	BREAKFAST	
	LUNCH	
	DINNER	
THURSDAY	BREAKFAST	
	LUNCH	
	DINNER	
FRIDAY	BREAKFAST	
	LUNCH	
	DINNER	
SARTURDAY	BREAKFAST	
	LUNCH	
	DINNER	
SUNDAY	BREAKFAST	
	LUNCH	
	DINNER	

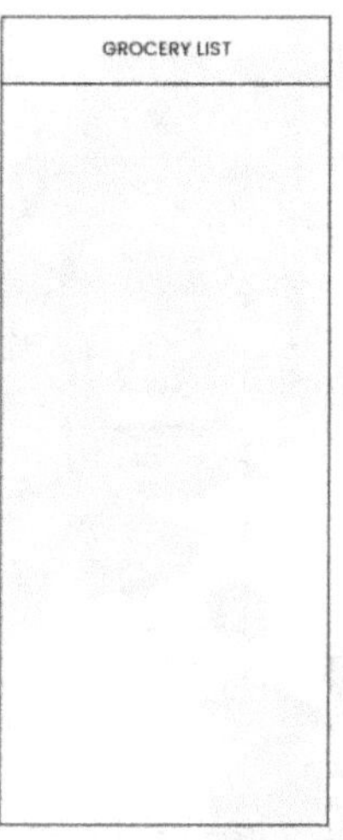

GROCERY LIST

SNACKS

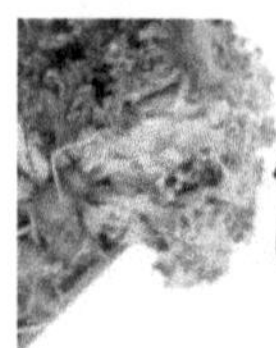

WEEKLY MEAL PLANNER

MONDAY	BREAKFAST	
	LUNCH	
	DINNER	
TUESDAY	BREAKFAST	
	LUNCH	
	DINNER	
WEDNESDAY	BREAKFAST	
	LUNCH	
	DINNER	
THURSDAY	BREAKFAST	
	LUNCH	
	DINNER	
FRIDAY	BREAKFAST	
	LUNCH	
	DINNER	
SARTURDAY	BREAKFAST	
	LUNCH	
	DINNER	
SUNDAY	BREAKFAST	
	LUNCH	
	DINNER	

GROCERY LIST

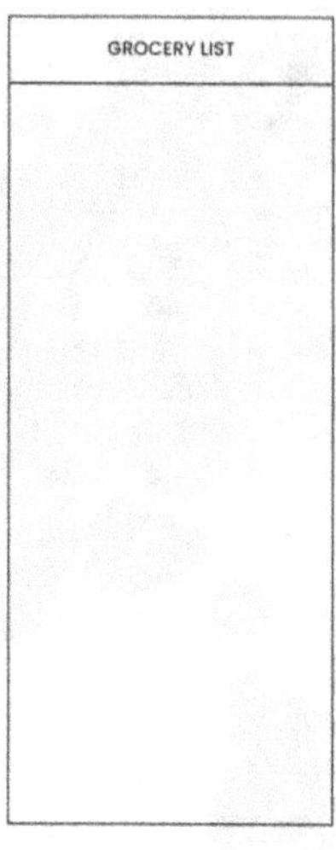

SNACKS

WEEKLY MEAL PLANNER

MONDAY	BREAKFAST	
	LUNCH	
	DINNER	
TUESDAY	BREAKFAST	
	LUNCH	
	DINNER	
WEDNESDAY	BREAKFAST	
	LUNCH	
	DINNER	
THURSDAY	BREAKFAST	
	LUNCH	
	DINNER	
FRIDAY	BREAKFAST	
	LUNCH	
	DINNER	
SARTURDAY	BREAKFAST	
	LUNCH	
	DINNER	
SUNDAY	BREAKFAST	
	LUNCH	
	DINNER	

GROCERY LIST

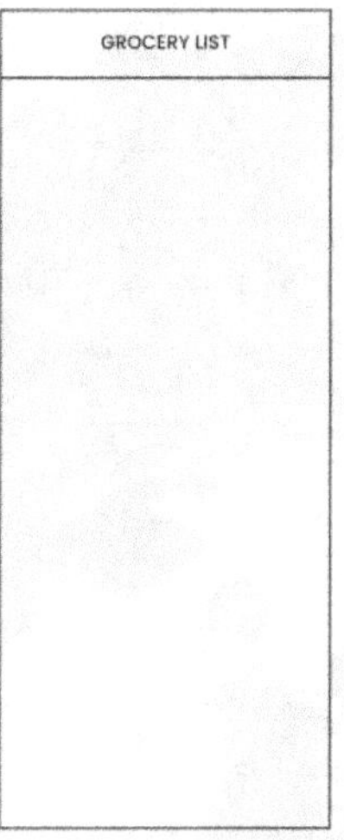

SNACKS

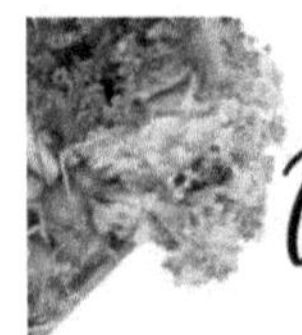

WEEKLY MEAL PLANNER

MONDAY	BREAKFAST	
	LUNCH	
	DINNER	
TUESDAY	BREAKFAST	
	LUNCH	
	DINNER	
WEDNESDAY	BREAKFAST	
	LUNCH	
	DINNER	
THURSDAY	BREAKFAST	
	LUNCH	
	DINNER	
FRIDAY	BREAKFAST	
	LUNCH	
	DINNER	
SARTURDAY	BREAKFAST	
	LUNCH	
	DINNER	
SUNDAY	BREAKFAST	
	LUNCH	
	DINNER	

GROCERY LIST

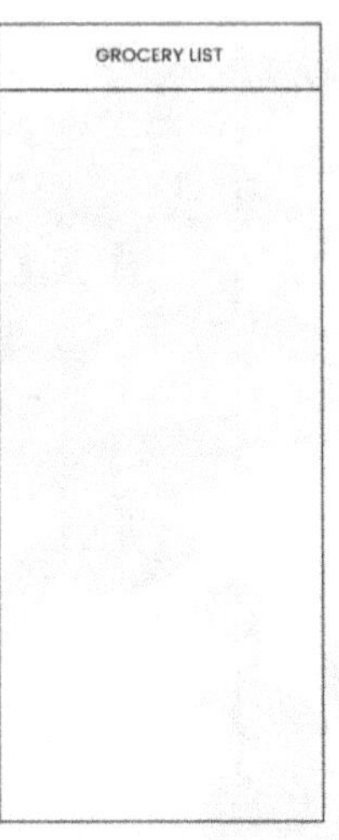

SNACKS

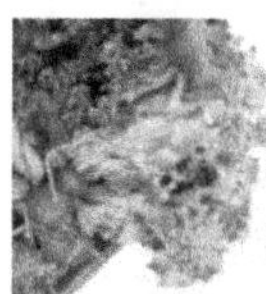

WEEKLY MEAL PLANNER

MONDAY	BREAKFAST	
	LUNCH	
	DINNER	
TUESDAY	BREAKFAST	
	LUNCH	
	DINNER	
WEDNESDAY	BREAKFAST	
	LUNCH	
	DINNER	
THURSDAY	BREAKFAST	
	LUNCH	
	DINNER	
FRIDAY	BREAKFAST	
	LUNCH	
	DINNER	
SARTURDAY	BREAKFAST	
	LUNCH	
	DINNER	
SUNDAY	BREAKFAST	
	LUNCH	
	DINNER	

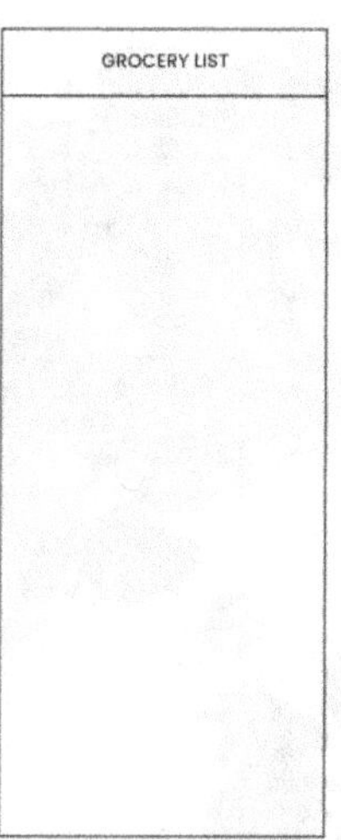

GROCERY LIST

SNACKS

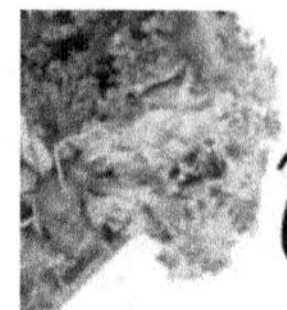

WEEKLY MEAL PLANNER

MONDAY	BREAKFAST	
	LUNCH	
	DINNER	
TUESDAY	BREAKFAST	
	LUNCH	
	DINNER	
WEDNESDAY	BREAKFAST	
	LUNCH	
	DINNER	
THURSDAY	BREAKFAST	
	LUNCH	
	DINNER	
FRIDAY	BREAKFAST	
	LUNCH	
	DINNER	
SARTURDAY	BREAKFAST	
	LUNCH	
	DINNER	
SUNDAY	BREAKFAST	
	LUNCH	
	DINNER	

GROCERY LIST

SNACKS

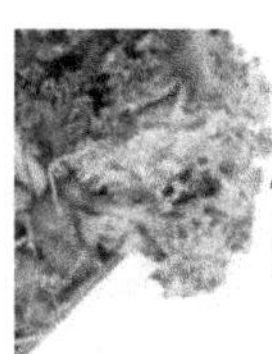

WEEKLY MEAL PLANNER

MONDAY	BREAKFAST	
	LUNCH	
	DINNER	
TUESDAY	BREAKFAST	
	LUNCH	
	DINNER	
WEDNESDAY	BREAKFAST	
	LUNCH	
	DINNER	
THURSDAY	BREAKFAST	
	LUNCH	
	DINNER	
FRIDAY	BREAKFAST	
	LUNCH	
	DINNER	
SARTURDAY	BREAKFAST	
	LUNCH	
	DINNER	
SUNDAY	BREAKFAST	
	LUNCH	
	DINNER	

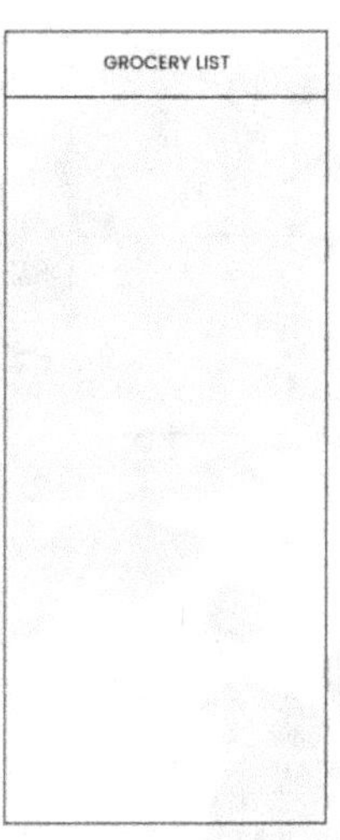

GROCERY LIST

SNACKS

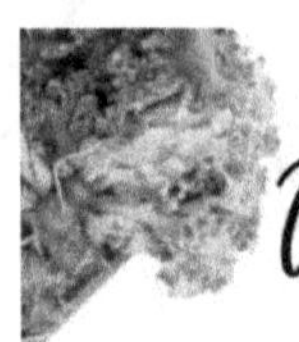

WEEKLY MEAL PLANNER

				GROCERY LIST
MONDAY	BREAKFAST			
	LUNCH			
	DINNER			
TUESDAY	BREAKFAST			
	LUNCH			
	DINNER			
WEDNESDAY	BREAKFAST			
	LUNCH			
	DINNER			
THURSDAY	BREAKFAST			
	LUNCH			
	DINNER			
FRIDAY	BREAKFAST			SNACKS
	LUNCH			
	DINNER			
SARTURDAY	BREAKFAST			
	LUNCH			
	DINNER			
SUNDAY	BREAKFAST			
	LUNCH			
	DINNER			

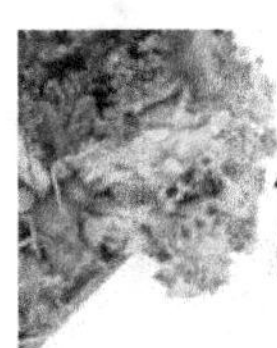

WEEKLY MEAL PLANNER

MONDAY	BREAKFAST		
	LUNCH		
	DINNER		
TUESDAY	BREAKFAST		
	LUNCH		
	DINNER		
WEDNESDAY	BREAKFAST		
	LUNCH		
	DINNER		
THURSDAY	BREAKFAST		
	LUNCH		
	DINNER		
FRIDAY	BREAKFAST		
	LUNCH		
	DINNER		
SARTURDAY	BREAKFAST		
	LUNCH		
	DINNER		
SUNDAY	BREAKFAST		
	LUNCH		
	DINNER		

GROCERY LIST

SNACKS

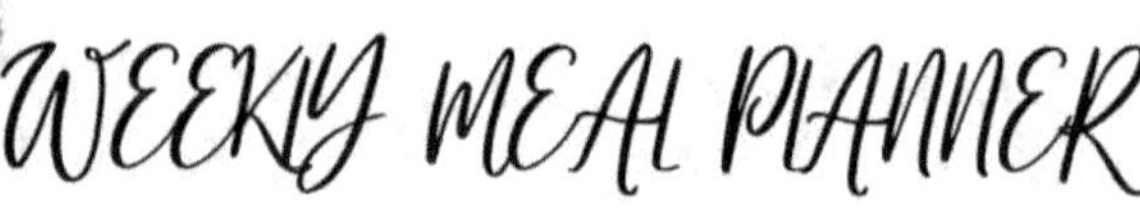

WEEKLY MEAL PLANNER

MONDAY	BREAKFAST	
	LUNCH	
	DINNER	
TUESDAY	BREAKFAST	
	LUNCH	
	DINNER	
WEDNESDAY	BREAKFAST	
	LUNCH	
	DINNER	
THURSDAY	BREAKFAST	
	LUNCH	
	DINNER	
FRIDAY	BREAKFAST	
	LUNCH	
	DINNER	
SARTURDAY	BREAKFAST	
	LUNCH	
	DINNER	
SUNDAY	BREAKFAST	
	LUNCH	
	DINNER	

GROCERY LIST

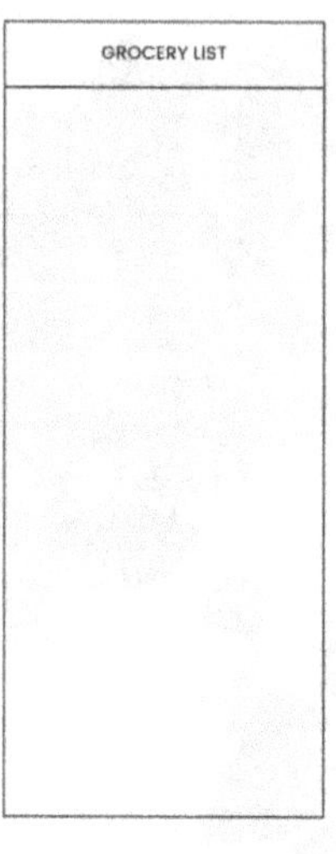

SNACKS

WEEKLY MEAL PLANNER

MONDAY	BREAKFAST	
	LUNCH	
	DINNER	
TUESDAY	BREAKFAST	
	LUNCH	
	DINNER	
WEDNESDAY	BREAKFAST	
	LUNCH	
	DINNER	
THURSDAY	BREAKFAST	
	LUNCH	
	DINNER	
FRIDAY	BREAKFAST	
	LUNCH	
	DINNER	
SARTURDAY	BREAKFAST	
	LUNCH	
	DINNER	
SUNDAY	BREAKFAST	
	LUNCH	
	DINNER	

GROCERY LIST

SNACKS

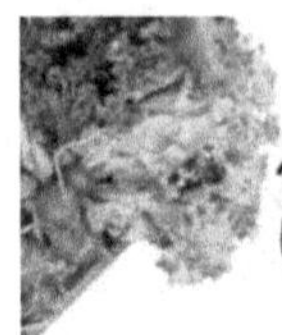

WEEKLY MEAL PLANNER

MONDAY	BREAKFAST	
	LUNCH	
	DINNER	
TUESDAY	BREAKFAST	
	LUNCH	
	DINNER	
WEDNESDAY	BREAKFAST	
	LUNCH	
	DINNER	
THURSDAY	BREAKFAST	
	LUNCH	
	DINNER	
FRIDAY	BREAKFAST	
	LUNCH	
	DINNER	
SARTURDAY	BREAKFAST	
	LUNCH	
	DINNER	
SUNDAY	BREAKFAST	
	LUNCH	
	DINNER	

GROCERY LIST

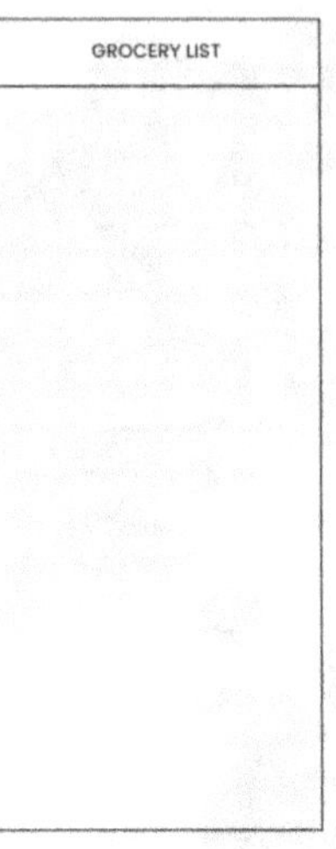

SNACKS

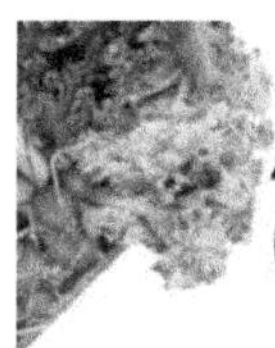

WEEKLY MEAL PLANNER

MONDAY	BREAKFAST	
	LUNCH	
	DINNER	
TUESDAY	BREAKFAST	
	LUNCH	
	DINNER	
WEDNESDAY	BREAKFAST	
	LUNCH	
	DINNER	
THURSDAY	BREAKFAST	
	LUNCH	
	DINNER	
FRIDAY	BREAKFAST	
	LUNCH	
	DINNER	
SARTURDAY	BREAKFAST	
	LUNCH	
	DINNER	
SUNDAY	BREAKFAST	
	LUNCH	
	DINNER	

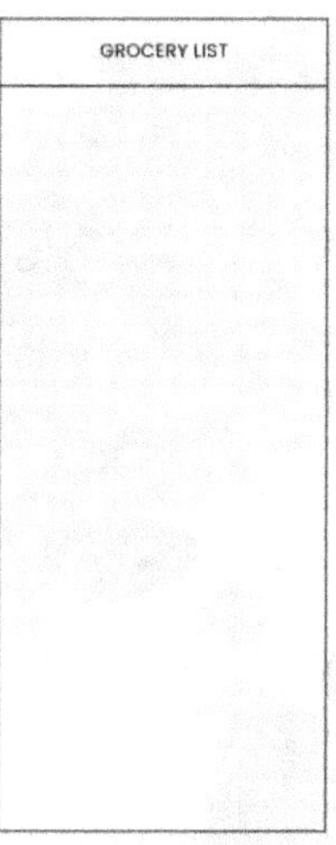

GROCERY LIST

SNACKS

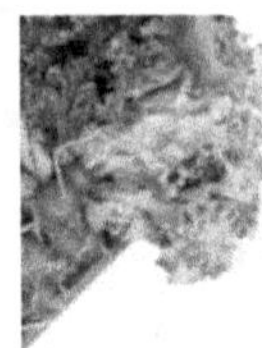

WEEKLY MEAL PLANNER

				GROCERY LIST
MONDAY	BREAKFAST			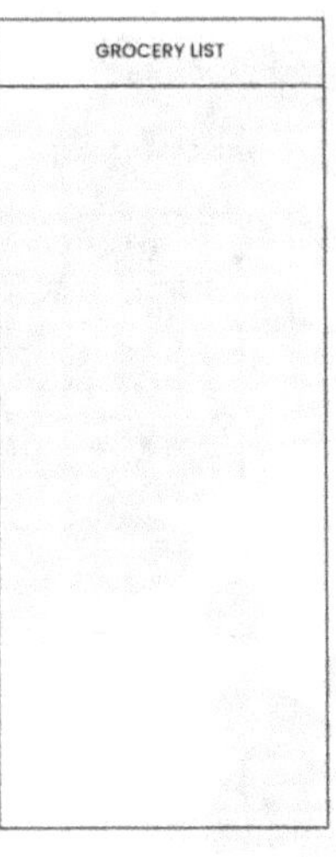
	LUNCH			
	DINNER			
TUESDAY	BREAKFAST			
	LUNCH			
	DINNER			
WEDNESDAY	BREAKFAST			
	LUNCH			
	DINNER			
THURSDAY	BREAKFAST			
	LUNCH			
	DINNER			
FRIDAY	BREAKFAST			SNACKS
	LUNCH			
	DINNER			
SARTURDAY	BREAKFAST			
	LUNCH			
	DINNER			
SUNDAY	BREAKFAST			
	LUNCH			
	DINNER			